# The Body-Mind Connection: Understanding the Pineal Gland's Impact on Wellbeing

Copyright Page

TITLE: The Body-Mind Connection: Understanding the Pineal Gland's Impact on Mental Wellbeing

1<sup>ST</sup> Edition

# Table of Contents


The Body-Mind Connection: Understanding the Pineal Gland's Impact on Mental Wellbeing...................................................................1

Chapter 1: Introduction to the Pineal Gland and its Impact on Mental Well-being........................................................................2

Chapter 2: Pineal Gland Detoxification Techniques ............................8

Chapter 3: Pineal Gland Activation through Meditation and Mindfulness ....................................................................... 15

Chapter 4: The Pineal Gland and its Role in Sleep and Circadian Rhythm Regulation ................................................................ 21

Chapter 5: The Pineal Gland and its Connection with Spiritual Awakening and Enlightenment ................................................. 27

Chapter 6: Pineal Gland Supplements and Natural Remedies for Enhancing its Function.................................................................. 33

Chapter 7: The Pineal Gland and its Relationship with Lucid Dreaming and Astral Projection ................................................... 38

Chapter 8: The Pineal Gland and its Significance in Ancient and Alternative Healing Practices .............................................. 44

Chapter 9: The Pineal Gland and its Role in Psychic Abilities and Intuition Development.................................................................. 51

Chapter 10: The Pineal Gland and its Association with the Third Eye Chakra and Energy Healing............................................... 58

Chapter 11: The Pineal Gland and its Impact on Mood, Emotions, and Mental Well-being ................................................................ 63

The Body-Mind Connection: Understanding the Pineal Gland's Impact on Mental Health

By Roberto Miguel Rodriguez

# Chapter 1: Introduction to the Pineal Gland and its Impact on Mental Well-being

The Significance of the Mind-Body Connection

The mind-body connection is a concept that has fascinated researchers, scientists, and spiritual practitioners for centuries. In recent years, there has been an increasing interest in understanding the role of the mind-body connection in promoting mental well-being. This subchapter explores the significance of this connection, focusing specifically on the pineal gland and its impact on our mental health.

The pineal gland, located deep within the brain, has long been associated with spiritual awakenings and enlightenment. It is often referred to as the "third eye" and is believed to be the gateway to higher consciousness. But its role extends beyond spirituality; the pineal gland also plays a crucial role in regulating our sleep patterns and circadian rhythms.

One of the most intriguing aspects of the mind-body connection is its association with psychic abilities and intuition development. Many ancient and alternative healing practices recognize the pineal gland as a key component in accessing these abilities. By enhancing the function of the pineal gland through meditation and mindfulness techniques, individuals can tap into their innate psychic potential and develop a deeper sense of intuition.

Furthermore, the pineal gland has a profound impact on our mood, emotions, and overall mental well-being. When the pineal gland is functioning optimally, it releases melatonin, a hormone that helps regulate sleep and mood. However, factors such as stress, environmental toxins, and a poor diet can disrupt the pineal gland's function, leading to imbalances in our mental and emotional states.

Fortunately, there are various techniques and natural remedies that can help detoxify and activate the pineal gland. From dietary changes to specific supplements, individuals can support the health and function of this vital gland. Moreover, practices like lucid dreaming and astral projection have been linked to the pineal gland, offering exciting opportunities for exploration and self-discovery.

Understanding the significance of the mind-body connection and the role of the pineal gland empowers individuals to take control of their mental well-being. By incorporating practices that enhance pineal gland function, such as meditation, mindfulness, and natural remedies, individuals can improve their sleep patterns, regulate their emotions, and tap into their innate spiritual potential.

In conclusion, the mind-body connection, specifically the role of the pineal gland, holds immense significance in promoting mental well-being. By exploring the various aspects of this connection, individuals can gain a deeper understanding of themselves and unlock their full potential for spiritual growth, psychic development, and emotional balance.

Understanding the Pineal Gland: An Overview

The pineal gland, a small endocrine gland located deep within the brain, has long been shrouded in mystery and intrigue. Often referred to as the "third eye" or the "seat of the soul," this tiny gland plays a vital role in our mental well-being and overall health. In this subchapter, we will explore the fascinating world of the pineal gland and gain a deeper understanding of its impact on our lives.

One of the key aspects we will delve into is the concept of pineal gland detoxification techniques. As we are exposed to an increasing number of toxins in our environment, it is crucial to learn how to cleanse and rejuvenate this vital gland. We will explore various methods and practices that can help us in this process, enabling us to optimize our mental well-being.

Furthermore, we will uncover the powerful connection between the pineal gland and meditation and mindfulness. By tapping into the potential of this gland, we can enhance our spiritual journey and achieve a higher state of consciousness. We will explore different techniques and practices that can activate the pineal gland, allowing us to experience a profound sense of peace and enlightenment.

Moreover, the pineal gland plays a significant role in regulating our sleep and circadian rhythms. We will examine the intricate relationship between this gland and our sleep patterns, exploring its impact on our ability to achieve restful sleep and maintain a healthy sleep-wake cycle. Understanding this connection can help us optimize our sleep and improve our overall well-being.

In addition, we will explore the pineal gland's role in spiritual awakening and enlightenment. Many ancient and alternative healing practices have recognized the pineal gland as a gateway to higher realms of consciousness. We will dive into the connection between the pineal gland and spiritual experiences, shedding light on how this gland can facilitate our journey towards self-discovery and spiritual growth.

Furthermore, we will discuss the significance of natural remedies and supplements in enhancing the function of the pineal gland. We will explore various herbs, vitamins, and minerals that can support the health of this gland and promote its optimal functioning.

Additionally, we will explore the pineal gland's association with lucid dreaming and astral projection. We will uncover how this gland can unlock the realms of the subconscious mind, enabling us to explore and navigate the dream world with clarity and intention.

Moreover, we will delve into the role of the pineal gland in ancient and alternative healing practices. From Ayurveda to Traditional Chinese Medicine, we will explore how different cultures have recognized the importance of this gland in achieving optimal health and well-being.

Furthermore, we will discuss the pineal gland's role in developing psychic abilities and intuition. We will explore how this gland acts as a receiver and transmitter of subtle energies, enabling us to tap into our innate intuitive abilities and enhance our psychic potential.

Lastly, we will examine the pineal gland's association with the third eye chakra and energy healing. We will explore how balancing and activating this energy center can lead to a deeper connection with our intuition, heightened awareness, and a greater sense of spiritual well-being.

In conclusion, the pineal gland is a remarkable and multifaceted organ that impacts various aspects of our mental well-being. By understanding its functions and exploring different techniques and practices, we can harness the power of this gland to optimize our overall health and enhance our spiritual journey.

The Link Between the Pineal Gland and Mental Health

The pineal gland, a small endocrine gland located deep within the brain, has long been a subject of fascination, mystery, and speculation. Often referred to as the "third eye," this tiny gland is believed to play a crucial role in our mental well-being, emotions, and overall mental health. In this subchapter, we will explore the intricate link between the pineal gland and mental health, shedding light on its various functions and how they impact our daily lives.

One of the key aspects we will delve into is the pineal gland's role in sleep and circadian rhythm regulation. This gland produces melatonin, a hormone that helps regulate our sleep-wake cycle. By understanding how the pineal gland controls our sleep patterns, we can gain insights into sleep disorders such as insomnia and develop effective strategies to improve our sleep quality.

Furthermore, we will explore the pineal gland's connection with spiritual awakening and enlightenment. Many spiritual traditions believe that the pineal gland is the gateway to higher consciousness and spiritual experiences. We will examine how practices like meditation and mindfulness can activate and awaken the pineal gland, leading to profound spiritual growth and an expanded sense of self.

Another intriguing aspect we will discuss is the pineal gland's association with psychic abilities and intuition development. Some studies suggest that a well-functioning pineal gland can enhance our intuitive abilities and psychic senses. We will explore various techniques and practices that can help us tap into this innate potential and cultivate our intuitive powers.

Moreover, we will explore the significance of the pineal gland in ancient and alternative healing practices. Throughout history, the pineal gland has been revered as a sacred organ in various cultures, with alternative healing modalities utilizing its energy and potential. We will delve into these practices and examine their impact on our mental well-being and overall health.

Lastly, we will discuss the role of the pineal gland in mood, emotions, and mental well-being. Research suggests that imbalances in the pineal gland can contribute to mood disorders such as depression and anxiety. By understanding the link between the pineal gland and our emotions, we can explore natural supplements and remedies that can enhance its function and promote emotional balance.

In conclusion, the pineal gland is a vital component of our mental health and well-being. By exploring its functions and understanding its impact on sleep, spirituality, intuition, ancient healing practices, and emotions, we can unlock its potential and harness its power to lead a more fulfilling and balanced life.

# Chapter 2: Pineal Gland Detoxification Techniques

The Importance of Detoxifying the Pineal Gland

In today's fast-paced and stressful world, maintaining optimal mental well-being is crucial. One often overlooked yet vital aspect of mental health is the pineal gland, a small gland located in the brain that plays a significant role in our overall well-being. Understanding the importance of detoxifying the pineal gland can offer valuable insights into enhancing mental health and achieving spiritual growth.

The pineal gland is responsible for producing melatonin, a hormone that regulates our sleep and wake cycles. However, due to various environmental factors, such as exposure to toxins, stress, and poor diet, the pineal gland can become calcified, hindering its proper function. This can result in sleep disturbances, mood swings, and a lack of mental clarity.

Detoxifying the pineal gland is crucial to restore its optimal function. There are various techniques available to achieve this, including dietary changes, meditation, and mindfulness practices. By adopting a clean and healthy diet, rich in antioxidants and essential nutrients, we can support the pineal gland's detoxification process. Additionally, incorporating meditation and mindfulness practices into our daily routine can help reduce stress and promote overall well-being, allowing the pineal gland to function optimally.

Furthermore, the pineal gland is often associated with spiritual awakening and enlightenment. Many ancient and alternative healing practices recognize the pineal gland as the "third eye" or the seat of intuition and psychic abilities. By detoxifying and activating the pineal gland, individuals can open themselves up to higher levels of consciousness, spiritual experiences, and a deeper connection with the universe.

Supplements and natural remedies can also aid in enhancing the pineal gland's function. Certain herbs, such as ashwagandha and holy basil, have been used for centuries to support the pineal gland and promote mental well-being. Additionally, incorporating practices like lucid dreaming and astral projection can help individuals explore their subconscious mind and tap into their hidden potential.

Moreover, the pineal gland's association with the third eye chakra and energy healing further emphasizes its significance in mental well-being. By balancing and harmonizing the energy flow in the body, individuals can experience improved mood, emotional stability, and a heightened sense of intuition.

In conclusion, understanding the importance of detoxifying the pineal gland is crucial for maintaining optimal mental well-being. By adopting various techniques such as dietary changes, meditation, and natural remedies, individuals can support the pineal gland's detoxification process and unlock its full potential. This can lead to improved sleep, enhanced spiritual experiences, and a greater sense of mental clarity and well-being.

Detoxification through Diet and Nutrition

In the quest for optimal mental well-being, it is crucial to address the health of the pineal gland, a small but mighty organ located deep within the brain. The pineal gland plays a pivotal role in regulating our sleep-wake cycles, known as circadian rhythms, as well as our mood, emotions, and overall mental well-being. One effective approach to support the pineal gland's function is through detoxification via diet and nutrition.

Toxins from our modern environment, such as heavy metals, pesticides, and synthetic chemicals, can accumulate in the pineal gland over time, impairing its ability to function optimally. This can lead to disruptions in sleep, mood imbalances, and a general sense of disconnection from our spiritual selves. However, by adopting a detoxifying diet, we can help cleanse and revitalize this vital organ.

The first step in pineal gland detoxification is to reduce or eliminate processed foods, which are often laden with artificial additives and preservatives. Instead, focus on consuming whole, organic foods that are rich in nutrients and antioxidants. Incorporate plenty of fresh fruits and vegetables, especially those high in vitamins A and C, such as leafy greens, berries, and citrus fruits. These powerful antioxidants help neutralize free radicals and protect the pineal gland from oxidative stress.

Additionally, it is important to limit exposure to fluoride, a mineral that can accumulate in the pineal gland and impair its function. Avoid consuming fluoridated water and opt for filtered or spring water instead. Green tea is also a great alternative to fluoride-laden beverages.

Furthermore, certain foods and herbs have been traditionally associated with enhancing pineal gland function. These include turmeric, which has potent anti-inflammatory properties, and raw cacao, which contains natural compounds that support the production of serotonin, a neurotransmitter involved in mood regulation.

To further support pineal gland detoxification, consider incorporating intermittent fasting into your routine. By giving your digestive system a break for a specific period of time, you allow your body to divert energy towards detoxification and repair processes.

In conclusion, detoxification through diet and nutrition is a powerful tool for supporting the health and vitality of the pineal gland. By adopting a clean, whole-foods diet, limiting exposure to toxins, and incorporating fasting, you can help cleanse and revitalize this remarkable organ, leading to improved sleep, mood, and overall mental well-being.

Detoxification through Lifestyle Changes

In today's fast-paced and highly stressful world, many of us are seeking ways to improve our mental well-being and find inner peace. One powerful tool that can help in this pursuit is detoxification through lifestyle changes. By making conscious choices about our daily habits and routines, we can support the health and function of the pineal gland, which in turn has a profound impact on our mental well-being.

The pineal gland, often referred to as the "third eye," is a small gland located deep within the brain. It plays a crucial role in regulating our sleep and circadian rhythm, which directly affects our overall mood, emotions, and mental well-being. However, due to various factors such as exposure to environmental toxins, poor diet, and chronic stress, the pineal gland can become calcified and its function compromised.

To detoxify the pineal gland and restore its optimal function, lifestyle changes are essential. One effective technique is to incorporate meditation and mindfulness practices into our daily routine. By taking the time to quiet the mind and focus our attention inward, we can activate the pineal gland and stimulate its function. Regular meditation has been shown to reduce stress, improve sleep quality, and enhance overall mental well-being.

In addition to meditation, there are various natural remedies and supplements that can support pineal gland health. These include herbs such as ashwagandha, holy basil, and chamomile, which have been used for centuries in ancient healing practices. These herbs help to reduce inflammation, promote detoxification, and enhance the function of the pineal gland.

Furthermore, lifestyle changes such as adopting a healthy diet and reducing exposure to environmental toxins can also support pineal gland detoxification. Consuming organic fruits and vegetables, limiting processed foods, and avoiding exposure to chemicals found in household products can all contribute to a healthier pineal gland.

The pineal gland is not only essential for regulating sleep and circadian rhythms but also has a deep connection with spiritual awakening and enlightenment. Many ancient healing practices, such as yoga and Ayurveda, recognize the pineal gland as a gateway to higher consciousness. By detoxifying and activating the pineal gland, individuals may experience heightened intuition, lucid dreaming, and even psychic abilities.

In conclusion, detoxification through lifestyle changes is a powerful method to enhance the function of the pineal gland and improve mental well-being. By incorporating practices such as meditation, mindfulness, and natural remedies, individuals can support the health of their pineal gland and experience a deeper sense of peace, clarity, and spiritual connection. In our hectic modern lives, taking the time to nurture and detoxify the pineal gland can be a transformative journey towards optimal mental and emotional well-being.

Other Detoxification Techniques

In addition to the well-known detoxification methods such as diet and exercise, there are several other techniques that can help in the detoxification of the pineal gland. The pineal gland, often referred to as the "third eye," plays a crucial role in our mental well-being and overall health. By incorporating these techniques into your daily routine, you can promote the activation and optimal functioning of this powerful gland.

One such technique is the practice of visualization. Visualization involves creating mental images that promote relaxation and healing. By visualizing a bright light shining on your pineal gland, you can stimulate its detoxification process. This technique is particularly effective when combined with deep breathing exercises, as it helps to oxygenate the pineal gland and enhance its function.

Another powerful technique is sound therapy. Certain frequencies and vibrations have been found to have a profound impact on the pineal gland. By listening to specific sound frequencies, such as binaural beats or Tibetan singing bowls, you can activate and cleanse the pineal gland. These frequencies help to release any blockages or toxins that may have accumulated in the gland, promoting mental clarity and emotional well-being.

Meditation and mindfulness practices are also highly effective in detoxifying the pineal gland. By quieting the mind and focusing on the present moment, you can reduce stress and promote the activation of the pineal gland. Regular meditation and mindfulness practices have been shown to enhance the production of melatonin, a hormone produced by the pineal gland that regulates sleep and circadian rhythms. By incorporating these practices into your daily routine, you can improve sleep quality and overall mental well-being.

In addition to these techniques, there are various natural remedies and supplements that can enhance the function of the pineal gland. Herbs such as ashwagandha, ginkgo biloba, and spirulina have been found to support pineal gland health and detoxification. These natural remedies can be incorporated into your diet or taken as supplements to promote optimal pineal gland function.

It is important to note that detoxifying the pineal gland is not a one-time process but a continuous practice. By incorporating these techniques into your daily routine, you can support the health and well-being of your pineal gland and unlock its full potential. As you embark on this journey, you may also experience an increased connection with your spirituality, heightened intuition, and a greater sense of inner peace and clarity. So, take the time to explore these detoxification techniques and unlock the power of your pineal gland for a healthier and more fulfilling life.

# Chapter 3: Pineal Gland Activation through Meditation and Mindfulness

The Power of Meditation in Activating the Pineal Gland

Meditation has been practiced for centuries as a way to calm the mind, reduce stress, and achieve a state of inner peace. However, its benefits extend far beyond these immediate effects. One area where meditation has shown significant impact is in activating the pineal gland, a small endocrine gland located deep within the brain.

The pineal gland, often referred to as the "third eye," plays a crucial role in regulating our sleep-wake cycle and circadian rhythm. It produces melatonin, a hormone that helps us fall asleep and stay asleep. By practicing meditation regularly, we can enhance the functioning of the pineal gland, leading to improved sleep quality and overall well-being.

Furthermore, meditation has long been associated with spiritual awakening and enlightenment. The pineal gland is believed to be the gateway to higher consciousness, and by activating it, we can access deeper levels of awareness and insight. Through mindfulness practices and focused meditation techniques, we can tap into the pineal gland's potential and experience profound spiritual growth.

Many individuals are interested in detoxifying their pineal gland, as it can become calcified over time due to factors such as fluoride exposure and a poor diet. Meditation offers a natural and effective way to cleanse and rejuvenate this vital gland. By quieting the mind and allowing our awareness to expand, we create an optimal environment for the pineal gland to release accumulated toxins and function at its highest potential.

In addition to meditation, there are various supplements and natural remedies available that can enhance the pineal gland's function. These include herbs like ashwagandha, turmeric, and ginkgo biloba, which have been used for centuries in ancient healing practices. However, it is important to consult with a healthcare professional before incorporating any new supplements into your routine.

The pineal gland is also closely linked to lucid dreaming and astral projection, two phenomena that involve conscious awareness during sleep. Through meditation and specific visualization techniques, we can train our minds to enter these states more easily and explore the depths of our subconscious.

Moreover, the pineal gland has been revered in ancient and alternative healing practices for its role in energy healing and balancing the chakras. By activating the pineal gland, we can unlock our intuitive abilities, enhance our psychic powers, and experience a deeper connection with the spiritual realm.

Finally, the pineal gland's impact on mood, emotions, and mental well-being should not be overlooked. When the pineal gland is functioning optimally, it helps regulate serotonin and other neurotransmitters, leading to improved mood and emotional stability. By incorporating meditation into our daily lives, we can support our pineal gland and promote a positive state of mind.

In conclusion, the power of meditation in activating the pineal gland is undeniable. Whether you are seeking better sleep, spiritual growth, or improved mental well-being, incorporating regular meditation practices into your routine can have transformative effects. By embracing the potential of the pineal gland, we can unlock new levels of consciousness and lead more fulfilling lives.

Mindfulness Practices for Pineal Gland Activation

In our fast-paced, modern world, it is becoming increasingly important to take care of our mental well-being. One often overlooked aspect of this is the pineal gland, a small gland located deep within our brain. The pineal gland plays a crucial role in regulating our sleep patterns, circadian rhythms, and even our spiritual awakening. In this subchapter, we will explore various mindfulness practices that can help activate and enhance the function of the pineal gland.

One of the most effective ways to activate the pineal gland is through meditation and mindfulness. By practicing mindfulness, we can train our minds to focus on the present moment, bringing awareness to the sensations in our body and the thoughts in our mind. This heightened state of awareness can help stimulate the pineal gland and promote its optimal functioning.

Another technique to consider for pineal gland activation is pineal gland detoxification. This involves adopting a clean and healthy lifestyle, free from toxins and harmful substances. By avoiding processed foods, artificial additives, and excessive alcohol or drug consumption, we can support the detoxification process of the pineal gland and promote its overall well-being.

Furthermore, the pineal gland has a deep connection with our spiritual awakening and enlightenment. By practicing mindfulness and engaging in spiritual practices such as yoga or energy healing, we can awaken the dormant potential of the pineal gland, known as the third eye. This can lead to heightened intuition, psychic abilities, and a greater sense of connection to the universe.

There are also natural remedies and supplements that can enhance the function of the pineal gland. Certain herbs, such as ashwagandha and holy basil, have been traditionally used to support the pineal gland's health and function. Additionally, melatonin supplements can help regulate sleep patterns and support the pineal gland's role in circadian rhythm regulation.

The pineal gland's impact on mood, emotions, and mental well-being should not be underestimated. By adopting mindfulness practices and incorporating them into our daily routine, we can cultivate a sense of inner peace, reduce stress, and improve our overall mental well-being. These practices can include breathing exercises, body scans, and mindful movement such as yoga or tai chi.

In conclusion, the pineal gland is a fascinating and important organ that plays a vital role in our mental well-being. By incorporating mindfulness practices into our lives, we can activate and enhance the function of the pineal gland, leading to improved sleep, spiritual awakening, and a greater sense of overall well-being. So, take a moment to breathe, be present, and nurture your pineal gland for a healthier mind-body connection.

Techniques for Cultivating Inner Awareness

In the pursuit of overall well-being and a deeper understanding of the mind-body connection, it is essential to cultivate inner awareness. This subchapter explores various techniques that can help individuals connect with their inner selves, harness the power of the pineal gland, and enhance their mental well-being.

One technique for cultivating inner awareness is pineal gland detoxification. By eliminating toxins and harmful substances from our bodies, we can optimize the functioning of the pineal gland. This can be achieved through dietary changes, such as reducing processed foods and increasing the intake of organic fruits and vegetables. Additionally, avoiding exposure to artificial light, electromagnetic radiation, and fluoride can aid in detoxification.

Meditation and mindfulness practices are powerful tools for activating the pineal gland. Regular meditation helps quiet the mind, reduce stress, and increase focus. By incorporating mindfulness into daily activities, individuals can cultivate present-moment awareness and develop a deeper connection with their inner selves.

The pineal gland plays a crucial role in regulating sleep and circadian rhythms. Techniques such as maintaining a consistent sleep schedule, creating a sleep-friendly environment, and practicing relaxation techniques before bed can support optimal pineal gland function and promote restful sleep.

Spiritual awakening and enlightenment are often associated with the pineal gland. Practices such as yoga, breathwork, and energy healing can stimulate the pineal gland and facilitate spiritual growth. Engaging in activities that promote self-reflection, such as journaling or spending time in nature, can also deepen one's spiritual connection.

Supplements and natural remedies can enhance the function of the pineal gland. Substances like melatonin, magnesium, and certain herbs have been found to support pineal gland health and promote overall well-being. However, it is important to consult with a healthcare professional before incorporating any supplements into your routine.

The pineal gland has been linked to lucid dreaming and astral projection. Techniques like dream journaling, reality checks, and specific meditation practices can increase dream recall and facilitate lucid dreaming. Exploring astral projection techniques can also provide individuals with profound spiritual experiences.

Ancient and alternative healing practices often recognize the significance of the pineal gland. Modalities such as acupuncture, Ayurveda, and sound healing can help balance the energy centers in the body, including the pineal gland, promoting overall health and well-being.

The pineal gland is believed to be connected to psychic abilities and intuition development. Techniques such as developing a regular meditation practice, practicing mindfulness, and engaging in energy healing modalities can enhance intuitive abilities and foster a deeper connection with one's inner wisdom.

The pineal gland is closely associated with the third eye chakra, an energy center located in the middle of the forehead. Balancing this chakra through meditation, visualization, and energy healing practices can promote clarity, intuition, and spiritual growth.

Finally, the pineal gland's impact on mood, emotions, and mental well-being cannot be overlooked. By implementing the techniques discussed in this subchapter, individuals can experience improved mental health, increased emotional resilience, and a greater sense of overall well-being.

In conclusion, cultivating inner awareness is vital for harnessing the power of the pineal gland and enhancing mental well-being. By incorporating techniques such as pineal gland detoxification, meditation and mindfulness practices, and exploring the pineal gland's connection to various aspects of life, individuals can embark on a transformative journey toward self-discovery and improved mental health.

# Chapter 4: The Pineal Gland and its Role in Sleep and Circadian Rhythm Regulation

Understanding Sleep and Circadian Rhythms

Sleep is a vital component of our overall well-being, yet many of us struggle to achieve a good night's rest. Have you ever wondered why some nights you effortlessly drift off to sleep, while on others, you toss and turn for hours? The answer lies in our body's internal clock, known as the circadian rhythm, which is regulated by a small, pinecone-shaped gland called the pineal gland.

The pineal gland, located deep within the brain, plays a crucial role in the regulation of our sleep-wake cycle. It produces a hormone called melatonin, which helps signal our body when it's time to sleep and wake up. Melatonin production is influenced by external factors such as light and darkness, which is why exposure to bright lights or screens before bed can disrupt our sleep patterns.

Understanding the pineal gland's role in sleep and circadian rhythm regulation opens up a world of possibilities for improving our sleep quality. By incorporating pineal gland detoxification techniques into our daily routine, we can help cleanse and rejuvenate this important gland. Practices such as dry brushing, consuming antioxidant-rich foods, and avoiding fluoride can all contribute to a healthier pineal gland.

Additionally, pineal gland activation through meditation and mindfulness has been shown to enhance our overall well-being. By practicing mindfulness and directing our attention inward, we can tap into the power of the pineal gland, leading to a more profound sense of peace, clarity, and spiritual awakening.

In ancient and alternative healing practices, the pineal gland has long been revered for its significance. It is often associated with the third eye chakra, which represents our intuition and connection to higher realms of consciousness. By exploring techniques such as energy healing and working with the pineal gland, we can deepen our spiritual journey and unlock hidden potentials within ourselves.

For those interested in enhancing the function of their pineal gland, natural remedies and supplements can be beneficial. Substances like ashwagandha, turmeric, and magnesium have been shown to support pineal gland health and promote better sleep quality.

Furthermore, the pineal gland's impact extends beyond sleep and spiritual awakening. It also influences our mood, emotions, and overall mental well-being. When our pineal gland is functioning optimally, we experience greater emotional stability, improved focus, and a more positive outlook on life.

The pineal gland's connection with lucid dreaming and astral projection is another intriguing area of study. By nurturing our pineal gland, we can potentially unlock the ability to control our dreams and explore astral planes, leading to profound experiences and personal growth.

In conclusion, understanding the role of the pineal gland in sleep and circadian rhythm regulation opens up a world of possibilities for improving our overall well-being. By incorporating techniques such as detoxification, activation through meditation, and exploring its connection with spirituality and ancient healing practices, we can enhance our sleep quality, tap into our intuition, and unlock hidden potentials within ourselves. Additionally, natural remedies, supplements, and exploring its impact on lucid dreaming and emotional well-being offer further avenues for exploration. Embracing the power of the pineal gland can lead to a more fulfilling and enlightened life.

The Pineal Gland's Role in Melatonin Production

The pineal gland, a small pea-sized gland located deep within the brain, plays a crucial role in melatonin production. Melatonin, often referred to as the "sleep hormone," is responsible for regulating our sleep-wake cycle and maintaining a healthy circadian rhythm.

The pineal gland produces melatonin in response to darkness and is suppressed by light. As the sun sets and darkness falls, the pineal gland begins to release melatonin into the bloodstream, signaling to the body that it is time to sleep. This natural process helps us fall asleep and stay asleep throughout the night.

Melatonin production is not only influenced by external factors such as light, but it is also affected by our internal state of well-being. Stress, anxiety, and other mental health issues can disrupt the pineal gland's ability to produce melatonin efficiently, leading to sleep disturbances and insomnia.

Understanding the pineal gland's role in melatonin production is essential for individuals seeking to improve their sleep quality and overall mental well-being. There are various techniques and practices that can enhance the functioning of the pineal gland and promote melatonin production.

One such technique is pineal gland detoxification, which involves adopting a healthy lifestyle and eliminating toxins from our environment and diet. By reducing exposure to environmental toxins, consuming a nutrient-rich diet, and practicing regular exercise, we can support the pineal gland's natural functions.

Meditation and mindfulness are powerful tools for activating the pineal gland. Through these practices, we can quiet the mind, reduce stress, and stimulate the pineal gland's secretion of melatonin. By incorporating meditation and mindfulness into our daily routine, we can improve both our sleep quality and overall mental well-being.

In addition to sleep regulation, the pineal gland is also associated with spiritual awakening and enlightenment. Many ancient and alternative healing practices, such as Ayurveda and yoga, recognize the pineal gland as the "third eye" or the seat of intuition and higher consciousness. By nurturing and activating the pineal gland, individuals can deepen their spiritual experiences and enhance their intuition.

Supplements and natural remedies can also be used to enhance the pineal gland's function. Substances like melatonin, magnesium, and certain herbs have been found to support the pineal gland's production of melatonin and promote restful sleep.

Furthermore, the pineal gland has been linked to lucid dreaming and astral projection. Lucid dreaming is the ability to become aware and control our dreams, while astral projection refers to the out-of-body experiences. By exploring and understanding the pineal gland's role in these phenomena, individuals can unlock new realms of consciousness and expand their spiritual journey.

Overall, the pineal gland's role in melatonin production extends far beyond regulating our sleep-wake cycle. It is intimately connected to our mental well-being, spiritual growth, and overall quality of life. By exploring the various techniques, practices, and remedies associated with the pineal gland, individuals can harness its power and unlock their true potential.

How to Optimize Sleep and Circadian Rhythms for Mental Well-being

Sleep plays a vital role in our overall mental well-being, and the pineal gland has a significant impact on regulating our sleep patterns and circadian rhythms. Understanding how to optimize sleep and circadian rhythms can greatly enhance our mental well-being. In this chapter, we will explore various techniques and practices that can help us achieve better sleep and improved mental health.

One important aspect of optimizing sleep is detoxifying the pineal gland. The pineal gland can accumulate toxins over time, which can interfere with its proper functioning. By adopting pineal gland detoxification techniques such as avoiding fluoride in water and toothpaste, reducing exposure to electronic devices before bed, and incorporating natural detoxifying foods into our diet, we can support the health of our pineal gland and promote better sleep.

Another powerful way to activate the pineal gland and improve sleep is through meditation and mindfulness. By practicing mindfulness meditation, we can calm the mind, reduce stress, and enhance our ability to fall asleep and maintain a restful sleep throughout the night. Additionally, specific meditative techniques, such as focusing on the third eye chakra, can help activate the pineal gland and promote a deeper connection with our spiritual self.

The pineal gland plays a crucial role in regulating our sleep-wake cycles and circadian rhythms. By understanding its role and implementing healthy sleep habits, such as maintaining a consistent sleep schedule, creating a sleep-conducive environment, and establishing a relaxing bedtime routine, we can optimize our sleep and support the pineal gland in its natural functions.

Furthermore, the pineal gland has been associated with spiritual awakening and enlightenment. Many ancient and alternative healing practices recognize the importance of the pineal gland in accessing higher states of consciousness. By nurturing the pineal gland through meditation, mindful practices, and a healthy lifestyle, we can deepen our spiritual journey and experience a profound sense of connection and enlightenment.

Supplements and natural remedies can also be beneficial in enhancing the function of the pineal gland. Certain herbs, such as ashwagandha and chamomile, have been traditionally used to support sleep and pineal gland health. However, it is important to consult with a healthcare professional before starting any supplement regimen.

The pineal gland is also connected to lucid dreaming and astral projection. By cultivating a strong and healthy pineal gland, we can improve our ability to have vivid and lucid dreams, as well as explore the realms of astral projection.

In conclusion, optimizing sleep and circadian rhythms is crucial for our mental well-being. By implementing pineal gland detoxification techniques, practicing meditation and mindfulness, understanding the role of the pineal gland in sleep regulation, and exploring its connection with spiritual awakening and enlightenment, we can enhance our mental health and overall quality of life. Additionally, incorporating natural remedies, exploring lucid dreaming and astral projection, and recognizing the significance of the pineal gland in ancient and alternative healing practices can further support our journey towards optimal mental well-being.

# Chapter 5: The Pineal Gland and its Connection with Spiritual Awakening and Enlightenment

Exploring the Spiritual Significance of the Pineal Gland

The pineal gland, a tiny pea-sized gland located deep within the brain, has fascinated scientists, philosophers, and spiritual seekers for centuries. In recent years, research has begun to shed light on the pineal gland's physical functions, such as its role in regulating sleep and circadian rhythms. However, this mysterious gland also holds immense spiritual significance, connecting us to higher realms of consciousness and inner wisdom.

One aspect of the pineal gland that has captivated many is its association with spiritual awakening and enlightenment. Ancient traditions and spiritual practices have long revered the pineal gland as the "third eye" or the seat of the soul. It is believed to be the gateway to higher dimensions of reality, allowing us to access profound spiritual insights and experiences.

Meditation and mindfulness are powerful tools for activating the pineal gland and deepening our spiritual connection. By quieting the mind and turning inward, we can stimulate the pineal gland's activity and open ourselves to spiritual experiences. Many spiritual traditions incorporate specific techniques to activate and awaken the pineal gland, leading to heightened states of consciousness and spiritual growth.

The pineal gland's significance extends beyond the realm of spirituality. It plays a crucial role in regulating our sleep patterns and circadian rhythms. Disruptions in the pineal gland's function can lead to sleep disorders and imbalances in our overall well-being. Understanding the pineal gland's role in sleep and circadian rhythm regulation can help us develop strategies for improving our sleep quality and maintaining optimal mental and physical health.

Additionally, the pineal gland is closely associated with the third eye chakra, a key energy center in the body. Balancing and activating the third eye chakra can enhance our intuition, psychic abilities, and connection to higher realms of consciousness. Various ancient and alternative healing practices, such as Ayurveda and acupuncture, target the pineal gland to restore balance and promote overall well-being.

For those seeking to enhance the pineal gland's function, natural remedies and supplements can be beneficial. Certain herbs, such as ashwagandha and holy basil, have been traditionally used to support pineal gland health. Additionally, lifestyle practices like reducing exposure to artificial light and incorporating healthy sleep habits can optimize the pineal gland's function.

In conclusion, the pineal gland holds immense spiritual significance and plays a crucial role in our overall well-being. Understanding its functions, such as its impact on sleep, circadian rhythms, and spiritual awakening, can empower us to cultivate a deeper connection with ourselves and the universe. By exploring techniques such as meditation, natural remedies, and ancient healing practices, we can unlock the pineal gland's potential and enhance our mental, emotional, and spiritual well-being.

The Pineal Gland's Role in Consciousness Expansion

The pineal gland, a small endocrine gland located deep within the brain, has long been associated with spiritual and metaphysical experiences. Often referred to as the "third eye," this tiny gland holds a significant role in consciousness expansion. In this subchapter, we will explore the various aspects of the pineal gland's impact on mental well-being and its connection to spirituality.

One of the most fascinating aspects of the pineal gland is its ability to be activated through meditation and mindfulness practices. By quieting the mind and focusing inward, individuals can tap into the pineal gland's potential for heightened awareness and expanded consciousness. This activation not only leads to a deeper understanding of oneself but also opens the doors to spiritual awakening and enlightenment.

Additionally, the pineal gland plays a crucial role in regulating sleep and circadian rhythms. Known as the body's internal clock, the pineal gland produces melatonin, a hormone that helps regulate sleep-wake cycles. By understanding the pineal gland's function, individuals can optimize their sleep patterns, leading to improved mental well-being and overall health.

The pineal gland's connection with spiritual awakening and enlightenment goes beyond sleep regulation. Many ancient and alternative healing practices recognize the pineal gland as a gateway to higher states of consciousness. Techniques such as pineal gland detoxification and natural remedies can enhance its function, allowing individuals to access deeper levels of awareness and spiritual growth.

Furthermore, the pineal gland is closely associated with lucid dreaming and astral projection. Lucid dreaming is the ability to become consciously aware and control one's dreams, while astral projection refers to the out-of-body experiences during sleep. By harnessing the power of the pineal gland, individuals can explore these realms and expand their understanding of the universe.

The significance of the pineal gland extends to psychic abilities, intuition development, and energy healing. Many believe that a fully activated pineal gland can enhance psychic abilities, such as clairvoyance and telepathy, and facilitate the development of intuition. Moreover, the pineal gland's association with the third eye chakra, an energy center in the body, highlights its importance in energy healing practices.

Lastly, the pineal gland's impact on mood, emotions, and mental well-being cannot be overlooked. Imbalances in the pineal gland can lead to mood disorders, depression, and anxiety. By maintaining the health and function of the pineal gland through various techniques and natural supplements, individuals can experience improved mental well-being and emotional stability.

In conclusion, the pineal gland's role in consciousness expansion is multifaceted and profound. From its connection to spirituality and metaphysical experiences to its impact on sleep, psychic abilities, and mental well-being, this tiny gland holds immense potential for personal growth and understanding. By exploring techniques such as meditation, detoxification, and natural remedies, individuals can tap into the power of the pineal gland and embark on a transformative journey towards expanded consciousness and enlightenment.

Practices for Spiritual Awakening and Enlightenment

The journey towards spiritual awakening and enlightenment is a deeply personal and transformative experience. It requires a commitment to self-discovery, inner growth, and a connection to something greater than ourselves. In this subchapter, we will explore various practices that can aid in this journey, specifically focusing on the role of the pineal gland.

One effective technique for pineal gland detoxification is maintaining a healthy lifestyle. This includes consuming a balanced diet rich in antioxidants, avoiding processed foods and toxins, and staying hydrated. Regular exercise, such as yoga or qigong, can also help stimulate the pineal gland and enhance its function.

Meditation and mindfulness are powerful tools for activating the pineal gland. By quieting the mind and focusing on the present moment, we can access deeper states of consciousness and expand our awareness. Regular meditation practice can help to awaken the pineal gland, leading to spiritual insights and a greater sense of connection to the universe.

The pineal gland plays a crucial role in regulating our sleep and circadian rhythm. Establishing a consistent sleep schedule, creating a peaceful sleep environment, and minimizing exposure to artificial light before bedtime can optimize the pineal gland's function and promote restful sleep.

The pineal gland is closely linked to spiritual awakening and enlightenment. Many ancient spiritual traditions recognize the pineal gland as the "third eye" or the seat of intuition and higher consciousness. Through practices such as visualization, breathwork, and energy healing, we can activate and align the pineal gland with our spiritual journey.

Supplements and natural remedies can also enhance the function of the pineal gland. Substances like melatonin, tryptophan, and certain herbs, such as ashwagandha and ginkgo biloba, have been known to support pineal gland health and stimulate spiritual experiences.

The pineal gland is associated with lucid dreaming and astral projection, allowing us to explore realms beyond the physical plane. By practicing lucid dreaming techniques and astral projection exercises, we can tap into the potential of the pineal gland and expand our consciousness.

The significance of the pineal gland in ancient and alternative healing practices cannot be overstated. Many indigenous cultures have used plant medicines, rituals, and sound healing to activate the pineal gland and facilitate spiritual growth.

The pineal gland is also closely connected to psychic abilities and intuition development. By honing our intuition through practices like journaling, intuitive exercises, and psychic development courses, we can strengthen the connection between the pineal gland and our intuitive faculties.

Lastly, the pineal gland plays a vital role in our mood, emotions, and overall mental well-being. By nurturing our pineal gland through these practices, we can experience a greater sense of inner peace, joy, and emotional balance.

In conclusion, the practices for spiritual awakening and enlightenment are diverse and multifaceted. By incorporating techniques such as pineal gland detoxification, meditation, sleep regulation, and supplement support, we can awaken the potential of the pineal gland and embark on a transformative journey towards spiritual growth and enlightenment.

# Chapter 6: Pineal Gland Supplements and Natural Remedies for Enhancing its Function

Introduction to Pineal Gland Supplements

Welcome to the subchapter on "Introduction to Pineal Gland Supplements" from the book "The Mind-Body Connection: Understanding the Pineal Gland's Impact on Mental Well-being". In this section, we will explore the fascinating world of pineal gland supplements and their potential to enhance various aspects of our mental well-being.

The pineal gland, a tiny pinecone-shaped gland located deep within the brain, has long been associated with spiritual awakening, intuition, and higher states of consciousness. It plays a crucial role in regulating our sleep patterns and circadian rhythm, which in turn affects our overall health and well-being.

One way to support and enhance the function of the pineal gland is through the use of supplements. These natural remedies can help detoxify and activate the pineal gland, leading to improved mental clarity, spiritual growth, and emotional balance.

Pineal gland supplements often contain ingredients such as melatonin, a hormone produced by the pineal gland that regulates sleep-wake cycles. By supplementing with melatonin, individuals can improve their sleep quality and overcome insomnia or jet lag.

Additionally, certain herbs and nutrients like ashwagandha, turmeric, and magnesium have been found to support the pineal gland's function. These supplements may help reduce stress and anxiety, promote relaxation, and support overall mental well-being.

Furthermore, pineal gland supplements are believed to enhance spiritual experiences and facilitate the opening of the third eye chakra. Many individuals report increased intuition, lucid dreaming, and even astral projection when incorporating these supplements into their daily routine.

It is important to note that while pineal gland supplements can be beneficial, they should be used in conjunction with other holistic practices such as meditation and mindfulness. These practices help to activate and awaken the pineal gland, allowing for a deeper connection with our spiritual selves.

In ancient and alternative healing practices, the pineal gland has been revered as the seat of the soul and a gateway to higher realms of consciousness. By incorporating pineal gland supplements into our lives, we can tap into this ancient wisdom and unlock our full spiritual potential.

In conclusion, pineal gland supplements offer a natural and holistic approach to enhancing mental well-being, promoting spiritual growth, and improving sleep patterns. By understanding the significance of the pineal gland and its role in various aspects of our lives, we can make informed decisions about incorporating these supplements into our daily routines.

Natural Remedies for Pineal Gland Support

The pineal gland, a small endocrine gland located in the brain, plays a crucial role in our mental well-being and overall health. It regulates our sleep patterns, circadian rhythms, and even has connections to our spiritual awakening and intuition. In this subchapter, we will explore various natural remedies that can support the health and function of the pineal gland.

One effective way to support the pineal gland is through detoxification techniques. The accumulation of toxins in our bodies can impair the pineal gland's function. Toxins can come from environmental pollutants, processed foods, and even stress. Incorporating practices such as regular exercise, drinking plenty of water, and consuming a balanced, organic diet can help eliminate toxins and promote the health of the pineal gland.

Meditation and mindfulness are also powerful tools for activating the pineal gland. By quieting the mind and focusing our attention inward, we can stimulate the pineal gland and enhance its function. Regular meditation and mindfulness practices can help improve sleep quality, reduce stress, and promote overall mental well-being.

Speaking of sleep, the pineal gland plays a vital role in regulating our sleep patterns and circadian rhythms. To support its function, it is essential to establish a regular sleep schedule, create a sleep-friendly environment, and practice good sleep hygiene. Avoiding electronic devices before bed, creating a relaxing bedtime routine, and ensuring a dark, quiet room can help optimize the pineal gland's ability to regulate sleep.

The pineal gland is often associated with spiritual awakening and enlightenment. Practices such as yoga, breathwork, and spending time in nature can help activate the pineal gland and deepen our spiritual connection. These practices promote relaxation, self-awareness, and a greater sense of inner peace.

In addition to lifestyle practices, certain supplements and natural remedies can enhance the function of the pineal gland. Some popular options include melatonin, which supports sleep regulation, and herbs like ashwagandha and bacopa, known for their ability to nourish the pineal gland and support mental well-being.

The pineal gland is also closely connected to dreams, psychic abilities, and intuition. Practices like lucid dreaming and astral projection can help us explore the deeper realms of consciousness and tap into our intuitive abilities. Keeping a dream journal, practicing visualization techniques, and engaging in energy healing modalities can all contribute to enhancing the pineal gland's connection to these experiences.

In conclusion, the pineal gland is a fascinating gland that plays a significant role in our mental well-being and spirituality. By incorporating natural remedies such as detoxification techniques, meditation, sleep regulation, and supplements, we can support the health and function of the pineal gland, leading to improved mood, enhanced intuition, and a deeper connection to our spiritual selves.

Precautions and Considerations in Using Supplements and Remedies

When it comes to enhancing the function of the pineal gland, many individuals turn to supplements and natural remedies. While these can be beneficial, it is important to exercise caution and consider certain factors before incorporating them into your routine. This subchapter aims to provide you with essential precautions and considerations to ensure your safety and maximize the potential benefits.

First and foremost, it is crucial to consult with a healthcare professional before starting any new supplement or remedy regimen. They can assess your specific needs, existing health conditions, and evaluate potential interactions with medications you may be taking. This step is especially important for individuals with pre-existing medical conditions or those who are pregnant or breastfeeding.

Additionally, it is vital to research and select reputable brands when purchasing supplements. Look for products that are third-party tested and certified to ensure their quality, purity, and potency. This will help you avoid any potential contamination or misleading claims that may be present in lesser-known brands.

Furthermore, it is important to follow the recommended dosage instructions provided by the manufacturer or healthcare professional. Taking excessive amounts of supplements can lead to adverse effects and may even be counterproductive. Remember, moderation is key.

While supplements and remedies can support the pineal gland's function, they should not be solely relied upon. It is essential to adopt a holistic approach that includes lifestyle modifications, such as maintaining a balanced diet, engaging in regular exercise, and managing stress effectively. These practices work synergistically with supplements to optimize the overall well-being of both the mind and body.

Lastly, it is worth noting that supplements and remedies are not a substitute for professional medical advice or treatment. If you are experiencing persistent or severe symptoms related to the pineal gland or mental well-being, it is crucial to seek guidance from a qualified healthcare professional. They can provide you with a comprehensive evaluation, diagnosis, and personalized treatment plan tailored to your specific needs.

In conclusion, while supplements and remedies can be valuable tools in enhancing the function of the pineal gland, it is essential to exercise caution and consider various factors before incorporating them into your daily routine. Consulting with a healthcare professional, selecting reputable brands, following recommended dosages, and adopting a holistic approach are all crucial steps to ensure your safety and maximize the potential benefits. Remember, the pineal gland's impact on mental well-being is multifaceted, and a comprehensive approach is key to achieving optimal results.

# Chapter 7: The Pineal Gland and its Relationship with Lucid Dreaming and Astral Projection

Understanding Lucid Dreaming and Astral Projection

Lucid dreaming and astral projection are fascinating phenomena that have captivated the human imagination for centuries. In this subchapter, we will explore the relationship between these experiences and the pineal gland, shedding light on the mind-body connection and its impact on mental well-being.

The pineal gland, often referred to as the "third eye," is a small endocrine gland located deep within the brain. It has long been associated with spiritual awakening and enlightenment in ancient and alternative healing practices. The pineal gland plays a crucial role in regulating our sleep-wake cycles and circadian rhythms, making it a key player in our overall well-being.

One of the most intriguing connections between the pineal gland and lucid dreaming is the role it plays in dream initiation and awareness. Lucid dreaming is the ability to become consciously aware that you are dreaming while still in the dream state. Research suggests that the pineal gland may produce and release the neurotransmitter DMT (Dimethyltryptamine), which is believed to contribute to the vividness and intensity of dreams. By activating the pineal gland through meditation and mindfulness practices, individuals may enhance their ability to have lucid dreams and gain control over their dream experiences.

Similarly, astral projection, also known as out-of-body experiences, involves a sense of separating one's consciousness from the physical body and traveling in a non-physical realm. Some spiritual traditions believe that the pineal gland is the gateway to higher dimensions and spiritual realms, facilitating astral projection experiences. By understanding the pineal gland's role and learning various techniques, individuals can explore and develop their ability to engage in astral projection.

Moreover, the pineal gland's significance extends beyond the realms of dreaming and spiritual experiences. It is believed to be intimately connected with our intuition, psychic abilities, and the development of the third eye chakra. By nourishing and enhancing the pineal gland's function through natural remedies and supplements, individuals may unlock their intuitive potential and strengthen their psychic abilities.

Furthermore, the pineal gland's impact on mood, emotions, and mental well-being cannot be overlooked. Imbalances in the pineal gland have been associated with mood disorders, such as depression and anxiety. By understanding the pineal gland's role in mental well-being, individuals can explore various detoxification techniques and lifestyle practices to support its optimal functioning, ultimately promoting emotional balance and overall mental health.

In conclusion, understanding the intricate relationship between the pineal gland, lucid dreaming, and astral projection opens up a world of possibilities for personal growth, spiritual exploration, and mental well-being. By delving into the mysteries of the mind-body connection, we can unlock the potential of the pineal gland and harness its power to enhance our dream experiences, spiritual awakening, intuition, and overall mental well-being.

How the Pineal Gland Affects Dream States

Dreams have long fascinated humans, often acting as gateways to the mysterious realms of the unconscious mind. But have you ever wondered what role the pineal gland plays in shaping our dream states? In this subchapter, we will delve into the fascinating connection between the pineal gland and our dreams, exploring its impact on mental well-being and its significance in various aspects of our lives.

The pineal gland, a small pea-sized gland located in the center of the brain, has been referred to as the "seat of the soul" for centuries. Ancient civilizations and alternative healing practices recognized its importance and believed it to be the gateway to higher consciousness and spiritual awakening. Modern science has started to unveil the secrets of this enigmatic gland, shedding light on its multifaceted role in our lives.

One of the most intriguing connections between the pineal gland and dreams is its involvement in regulating sleep and circadian rhythms. The pineal gland produces melatonin, a hormone that helps regulate our sleep-wake cycles. When the pineal gland is functioning optimally, it ensures a restful and rejuvenating sleep, leading to vivid and meaningful dreams.

Furthermore, the pineal gland is closely associated with the third eye chakra, an energy center located in the middle of the forehead. This chakra is believed to be the seat of intuition and psychic abilities. Activating the pineal gland through meditation and mindfulness practices can enhance our intuitive abilities and enable us to tap into the hidden realms of consciousness.

Moreover, the pineal gland is not only connected to our sleep and spiritual experiences but also plays a crucial role in our overall mental well-being. Imbalances in the pineal gland have been linked to mood disorders, such as depression and anxiety. By understanding how to optimize the function of this gland, we can potentially improve our mental health and emotional well-being.

In this subchapter, we will explore various techniques for pineal gland detoxification, activation, and enhancement. We will delve into natural remedies and supplements that can support its proper functioning.

Additionally, we will investigate the pineal gland's association with lucid dreaming, astral projection, and its significance in ancient and alternative healing practices.

Whether you are seeking to enhance your dream experiences, tap into your intuitive abilities, or improve your mental well-being, understanding the pineal gland's role in dream states is essential. Join us on this captivating journey as we unravel the secrets of the pineal gland and its profound impact on our dreams, spirituality, and overall mental well-being.

Techniques for Enhancing Lucid Dreaming and Astral Projection

Lucid dreaming and astral projection have fascinated humans for centuries, offering a gateway to explore the realms beyond our physical reality. In this subchapter, we will delve into various techniques that can enhance these extraordinary experiences, all while harnessing the power of the pineal gland.

One of the most effective ways to enhance lucid dreaming and astral projection is by detoxifying the pineal gland. Over time, this small gland can become calcified due to the accumulation of toxins, hindering its function. By adopting pineal gland detoxification techniques such as consuming a healthy diet, reducing exposure to fluoride, and practicing intermittent fasting, we can cleanse and activate this vital gland.

Meditation and mindfulness play a crucial role in activating the pineal gland. Regular practice can help quiet the mind, allowing us to access altered states of consciousness. By focusing our awareness on the pineal gland during meditation, we can stimulate its function and deepen our connection with the spiritual realm.

Understanding the pineal gland's role in sleep and circadian rhythm regulation is essential for enhancing lucid dreaming and astral projection. By establishing a consistent sleep schedule, creating a soothing bedtime routine, and incorporating relaxation techniques like deep breathing and visualization, we can improve the quality of our sleep and increase the likelihood of lucid dreaming and astral projection.

Ancient and alternative healing practices also recognize the significance of the pineal gland. Techniques such as sound therapy, crystal healing, and energy work can help activate and balance this gland, leading to profound spiritual awakening and enlightenment.

Supplements and natural remedies can provide additional support for enhancing the pineal gland's function. Substances like melatonin, magnesium, and certain herbs like chamomile and passionflower have been shown to promote lucid dreaming and astral projection.

Developing psychic abilities and intuition are closely linked to the pineal gland. By practicing techniques such as visualization, dream journaling, and connecting with our higher self through meditation, we can strengthen our intuitive powers and tap into the limitless potential of the mind.

The pineal gland's association with the third eye chakra and energy healing is undeniable. By clearing and balancing the third eye chakra through practices like yoga, Reiki, and acupuncture, we can enhance the pineal gland's function and promote overall well-being.

Lastly, it is crucial to understand the profound impact of the pineal gland on mood, emotions, and mental well-being. Through its regulation of serotonin, melatonin, and other neurotransmitters, the pineal gland plays a vital role in maintaining emotional balance and supporting mental health.

In conclusion, by implementing these techniques for enhancing lucid dreaming and astral projection, we can unlock the full potential of the pineal gland and embark on incredible journeys of self-discovery and spiritual growth. The mind-body connection, facilitated by the pineal gland, holds the key to unlocking the mysteries of our consciousness and expanding our understanding of the universe.

# Chapter 8: The Pineal Gland and its Significance in Ancient and Alternative Healing Practices

Historical Perspectives on the Pineal Gland

The pineal gland, a small endocrine organ located deep within the brain, has fascinated philosophers, spiritual leaders, and scientists for centuries. In this subchapter, we will explore the historical perspectives surrounding the pineal gland, shedding light on its mystical and scientific significance.

Ancient civilizations, such as the Egyptians and Greeks, believed the pineal gland to be the seat of the soul and the gateway to higher consciousness. Renowned philosopher Descartes even referred to it as the "principal seat of the soul." These early beliefs attributed mystical and spiritual qualities to the pineal gland, recognizing its connection to intuition, psychic abilities, and spiritual awakening.

As scientific understanding advanced, the pineal gland's role in regulating sleep and circadian rhythms came to the forefront. Scientists discovered that this small gland secretes melatonin, a hormone that helps regulate sleep-wake cycles. This finding highlighted the pineal gland's crucial role in maintaining our body's internal clock and ensuring a healthy sleep pattern.

In recent years, interest in the pineal gland has surged within the fields of alternative medicine and spirituality. Meditation and mindfulness practices have been found to activate and awaken the pineal gland, leading to enhanced mental well-being and spiritual experiences. Many individuals have reported increased intuition, clarity of thought, and a deeper connection to their spiritual selves through these practices.

Furthermore, the pineal gland's association with the third eye chakra, an energy center in the body, has gained attention. Ancient healing practices, such as Ayurveda and Traditional Chinese Medicine, have long recognized the pineal gland's significance in balancing energy flow and promoting overall well-being.

Supplements and natural remedies have also emerged as tools to enhance pineal gland function. Various herbs and minerals, such as ashwagandha, gotu kola, and iodine, have been linked to supporting the pineal gland's health and optimizing its function.

Moreover, the pineal gland's impact on mood, emotions, and mental well-being cannot be overlooked. Imbalances in melatonin production, often associated with disrupted sleep patterns, have been linked to mood disorders such as depression and anxiety. Understanding the pineal gland's role in regulating these emotions can lead to novel therapeutic approaches and promote mental well-being.

In conclusion, the pineal gland's historical perspectives encompass a rich tapestry of mystical beliefs, scientific discoveries, and alternative healing practices. From its association with spiritual awakening to its role in sleep regulation and mental well-being, the pineal gland continues to captivate and inspire researchers, practitioners, and individuals seeking to unlock its potential for enhanced well-being and spiritual growth.

Ancient Healing Practices and the Pineal Gland

The pineal gland, often referred to as the "third eye," has long been revered in ancient healing practices for its profound impact on mental well-being. Throughout history, cultures worldwide have recognized the pineal gland's significance and sought various techniques to harness its power. This subchapter explores the deep connection between ancient healing practices and the pineal gland, shedding light on its role in enhancing overall health and spiritual growth.

One of the key aspects of ancient healing practices involves detoxification techniques to cleanse and rejuvenate the pineal gland. These practices aim to remove toxins and calcification that may hinder its optimal functioning. Incorporating natural remedies such as consuming organic foods, avoiding fluoride, and practicing intermittent fasting can support pineal gland detoxification.

Meditation and mindfulness have been central to activating and awakening the pineal gland. By quieting the mind and focusing inward, individuals can tap into the gland's inherent potential. Ancient spiritual traditions, such as yoga and qigong, employ specific postures, breathing exercises, and visualization techniques to stimulate the pineal gland and open the third eye.

The pineal gland also plays a vital role in regulating sleep patterns and circadian rhythms. Ancient healing practices recognize this connection and offer techniques to optimize sleep quality. Creating a conducive sleep environment, practicing relaxation techniques before bed, and following a consistent sleep schedule can help align the pineal gland with natural sleep-wake cycles, promoting restful sleep and overall well-being.

Many ancient cultures believe that the pineal gland is the gateway to spiritual awakening and enlightenment. By activating the pineal gland, individuals can access higher states of consciousness and connect with their inner divinity. Through practices such as meditation, energy healing, and sound therapy, individuals can expand their spiritual awareness and experience profound transformation.

In addition to these practices, various supplements and natural remedies can enhance the pineal gland's function. Herbs like ashwagandha, bacopa, and ginkgo biloba have been traditionally used to support pineal gland health and cognition. Incorporating these natural remedies into one's lifestyle can enhance mental clarity, focus, and overall mental well-being.

Furthermore, the pineal gland's association with lucid dreaming and astral projection has fascinated ancient healers for centuries. Techniques like dream journaling, reality checks, and lucid dreaming induction practices can help individuals access the realms of the subconscious mind, leading to personal growth and self-discovery.

The pineal gland's significance in ancient and alternative healing practices extends to its role in developing psychic abilities and intuition. By activating the pineal gland, individuals can heighten their intuition and tap into their innate psychic potential. Practices such as energy healing, chakra balancing, and divination can support the alignment of the pineal gland with higher consciousness.

Moreover, the pineal gland's association with the third eye chakra and energy healing practices underscores its importance in overall well-being. By keeping the pineal gland balanced and harmonized, individuals can experience improved mood, emotional stability, and mental clarity. Ancient healing modalities such as acupuncture, Reiki, and crystal therapy can support the optimal functioning of the pineal gland and promote holistic well-being.

In conclusion, ancient healing practices have long recognized the profound impact of the pineal gland on mental well-being. By incorporating techniques such as detoxification, meditation, sleep regulation, spiritual awakening, natural remedies, lucid dreaming, psychic development, and energy healing, individuals can unlock the pineal gland's immense potential. Understanding and embracing the pineal gland's role in ancient healing practices can empower individuals to cultivate a deeper connection to themselves and the world around them, leading to enhanced mental well-being and spiritual growth.

Alternative Healing Modalities and the Pineal Gland

The pineal gland is a small, pinecone-shaped gland located deep within the brain. While its primary function is still not fully understood, it has long been associated with various alternative healing modalities and spiritual practices. In this subchapter, we will explore the fascinating connection between the pineal gland and these alternative healing modalities, shedding light on its impact on mental well-being and overall health.

One aspect that has gained significant attention is pineal gland detoxification techniques. Many believe that toxins, such as fluoride and heavy metals, can accumulate in the pineal gland, hindering its optimal functioning. Various detoxification techniques, including dietary changes, herbal supplements, and specialized cleansing protocols, have been suggested to cleanse and rejuvenate the pineal gland. These techniques aim to promote clarity of mind, enhance intuition, and improve overall mental well-being.

Another avenue for activating the pineal gland is through meditation and mindfulness practices. By quieting the mind and focusing inward, individuals can stimulate the pineal gland and promote its optimal functioning. Meditation techniques, such as visualization and third eye-focused meditation, are believed to activate and awaken the pineal gland, leading to heightened spiritual experiences and a greater sense of connection with the universe.

The pineal gland also plays a crucial role in sleep and circadian rhythm regulation. It produces melatonin, a hormone that helps regulate sleep-wake cycles. Disruptions in the pineal gland's function can lead to sleep disorders, such as insomnia or disrupted circadian rhythms. Understanding the pineal gland's role in sleep and circadian rhythm regulation can help individuals optimize their sleep patterns and improve their overall mental well-being.

Moreover, the pineal gland has been linked to spiritual awakening and enlightenment. Many ancient and alternative healing practices, such as yoga and Ayurveda, recognize the pineal gland as the seat of spiritual consciousness. Activating and aligning the pineal gland is believed to open doors to higher states of consciousness, deepened intuition, and spiritual experiences. Exploring this connection can provide valuable insights into the path of spiritual growth and self-discovery.

For those seeking to enhance the function of their pineal gland, natural remedies and supplements can be beneficial. Certain herbs, such as ashwagandha and bacopa, are known for their potential to support pineal gland health. Additionally, nutritional supplements, such as vitamin D and omega-3 fatty acids, have been associated with improved pineal gland function. Understanding these natural remedies can empower individuals to take an active role in enhancing their mental well-being.

Furthermore, the pineal gland's association with lucid dreaming and astral projection is another intriguing aspect. Some believe that by stimulating the pineal gland, individuals can experience vivid and conscious dreams, enabling them to explore realms beyond the physical. Exploring the connection between the pineal gland and these extraordinary states of consciousness can open up new possibilities for personal growth and self-exploration.

The pineal gland's significance in ancient and alternative healing practices cannot be overstated. Throughout history, various cultures have recognized the pineal gland as the gateway to heightened spiritual awareness and healing abilities. Understanding these ancient practices and their connection to the pineal gland can provide valuable insights into alternative healing modalities and their potential impact on mental well-being.

In addition, the pineal gland is believed to play a role in psychic abilities and intuition development. Many individuals report heightened intuition and psychic experiences when their pineal gland is activated and aligned. Exploring the relationship between the pineal gland and these extraordinary abilities can help individuals tap into their innate intuitive powers and expand their consciousness.

Moreover, the pineal gland is closely associated with the third eye chakra and energy healing. The third eye chakra, located in the center of the forehead, is believed to be connected to the pineal gland. By balancing and harmonizing the third eye chakra, individuals can promote the optimal functioning of the pineal gland and enhance their energy healing abilities. Exploring this connection can provide insights into the profound interplay between the pineal gland, chakras, and energy healing practices.

Finally, the pineal gland's impact on mood, emotions, and mental well-being cannot be overlooked. Disruptions in the pineal gland's function have been associated with mood disorders, such as depression and anxiety. By understanding the pineal gland's role in regulating neurotransmitters and hormonal balance, individuals can take proactive steps to support their mental well-being and emotional stability.

As we delve into the fascinating world of alternative healing modalities and the pineal gland, we will uncover the profound impact this tiny gland has on our mental well-being and overall health. By exploring its connection with detoxification techniques, meditation and mindfulness practices, sleep regulation, spiritual awakening, natural remedies, lucid dreaming, ancient healing practices, psychic abilities, chakras, and emotional balance, we will empower ourselves to take an active role in optimizing our mental well-being and unlocking our full potential.

# Chapter 9: The Pineal Gland and its Role in Psychic Abilities and Intuition Development

Exploring Psychic Abilities and Intuition

The human mind is a fascinating and complex entity, capable of extraordinary feats beyond our normal perception. Within the realm of psychic abilities and intuition lies a vast potential waiting to be unlocked. In this subchapter, we will delve into the intriguing connection between the pineal gland and these extraordinary phenomena.

The pineal gland, often referred to as the "third eye," is a small endocrine gland located deep within the brain. This remarkable gland has long been associated with spiritual awakening, intuition, and psychic abilities. It is believed to be the gateway between the physical and spiritual realms, connecting us to higher consciousness.

One of the most effective ways to activate the pineal gland and enhance psychic abilities is through meditation and mindfulness practices. By quieting the mind and focusing our attention inward, we create a conducive environment for the pineal gland to awaken and function optimally. Regular meditation not only strengthens our intuition but also improves mental well-being and overall clarity of thought.

Furthermore, the pineal gland plays a crucial role in regulating our sleep patterns and circadian rhythms. It produces melatonin, a hormone that helps us maintain a healthy sleep-wake cycle. When our pineal gland is functioning optimally, we experience restful sleep, vivid dreams, and even the potential for lucid dreaming and astral projection.

Ancient cultures and alternative healing practices have recognized the significance of the pineal gland for centuries. Practices such as yoga, Reiki, and energy healing aim to balance and activate the pineal gland, leading to spiritual growth and enlightenment. Additionally, various supplements and natural remedies, such as melatonin, ginkgo biloba, and certain herbs, can help enhance the function of the pineal gland.

The pineal gland's association with the third eye chakra further highlights its role in psychic development. Opening and balancing the third eye chakra can lead to heightened intuition, increased clarity, and a deeper connection to our inner wisdom. Energy healing modalities, such as chakra balancing and crystal therapy, can help stimulate and align the third eye chakra, supporting the pineal gland's function.

It is important to note that the pineal gland's impact extends beyond the realm of spirituality and psychic abilities. Research suggests that imbalances in the pineal gland may contribute to mood disorders, such as depression and anxiety. By nurturing and supporting this vital gland, we can experience improved mood, emotional well-being, and mental clarity.

In conclusion, the pineal gland holds immense potential for unlocking our psychic abilities and intuition. Through various techniques, such as meditation, mindfulness, energy healing, and supplementation, we can activate and enhance the function of this remarkable gland. By cultivating a deeper connection with our pineal gland, we can awaken the hidden powers of our mind and experience a profound transformation in our mental well-being and spiritual journey.

The Pineal Gland's Connection to Psychic Perception

The pineal gland, often referred to as the "third eye," has long been associated with psychic abilities and intuition. In this subchapter, we will explore the fascinating connection between the pineal gland and psychic perception, shedding light on the mysteries surrounding this enigmatic gland.

One of the most intriguing aspects of the pineal gland is its role in spiritual awakening and enlightenment. Many spiritual traditions believe that the pineal gland is the gateway to higher consciousness and spiritual realms. It is said to act as a receiver and transmitter of spiritual energy, allowing individuals to tap into their psychic abilities and access information beyond the physical realm.

To enhance the pineal gland's function and promote psychic perception, various techniques can be employed. Pineal gland detoxification techniques, such as avoiding fluoride and heavy metals, can help remove harmful substances that may inhibit its optimal functioning. Additionally, meditation and mindfulness practices have been found to activate the pineal gland, facilitating a deeper connection to one's intuition and psychic abilities.

The pineal gland's impact on sleep and circadian rhythm regulation is another crucial aspect to consider. As the gland responsible for producing melatonin, a hormone that regulates sleep-wake cycles, any imbalance in its function can disrupt sleep patterns and affect overall mental well-being. By maintaining a healthy pineal gland through lifestyle choices, such as getting regular exposure to natural light and avoiding artificial light at night, individuals can improve their sleep quality and enhance their psychic abilities.

Ancient and alternative healing practices have long recognized the significance of the pineal gland. From Ayurveda to Chinese medicine, various modalities incorporate techniques to activate and balance the pineal gland, promoting overall well-being. Similarly, the association between the pineal gland and the third eye chakra, a powerful energy center, highlights the gland's role in energy healing and psychic development.

For those looking to enhance their psychic abilities, natural remedies and supplements can be beneficial. Certain herbs, such as ashwagandha and gotu kola, are known to support pineal gland function and promote intuition. However, it is crucial to consult with a healthcare professional before incorporating any supplements into your routine.

Furthermore, the pineal gland's impact on mood, emotions, and mental well-being cannot be overlooked. Imbalances in the gland's function have been associated with depression, anxiety, and other mental health conditions. By nurturing the pineal gland through mindfulness practices, proper sleep hygiene, and a healthy lifestyle, individuals can improve their mental well-being and unlock their psychic potential.

In conclusion, the pineal gland's connection to psychic perception is a topic of great interest and significance. The understanding of this connection opens up new avenues for exploring our spiritual potential and deepening our intuition. By incorporating pineal gland detoxification techniques, meditation and mindfulness practices, and natural remedies, individuals can enhance their psychic abilities and experience a profound transformation in their mental well-being.

Techniques for Developing Psychic Abilities and Intuition

The human mind possesses incredible potential, including the ability to tap into psychic abilities and intuition. Developing these skills can provide valuable insights, heightened awareness, and a deeper connection with the world around us. In this subchapter, we will explore various techniques that can help unlock and enhance psychic abilities and intuition, all of which are influenced by the powerful pineal gland.

Pineal Gland Detoxification Techniques:

To optimize the functioning of the pineal gland, it is crucial to maintain its health and vitality. Detoxification practices such as avoiding fluoride and other toxins, consuming a balanced diet rich in antioxidants, and engaging in regular exercise can help cleanse and rejuvenate the pineal gland.

Pineal Gland Activation through Meditation and Mindfulness:

Meditation and mindfulness practices have long been associated with activating and awakening the pineal gland. By quieting the mind, focusing on the present moment, and directing our attention inward, we can access the pineal gland's latent potential and open the gateway to psychic abilities and intuition.

Pineal Gland and its Role in Sleep and Circadian Rhythm Regulation:

The pineal gland plays a vital role in regulating our sleep-wake cycles and circadian rhythms. By establishing a consistent sleep routine, minimizing exposure to artificial light before bed, and creating a peaceful sleep environment, we can support the pineal gland's optimal function and enhance our psychic abilities and intuition.

Pineal Gland and its Connection with Spiritual Awakening and Enlightenment:

The pineal gland is often referred to as the "seat of the soul" due to its connection with spiritual experiences. By engaging in spiritual practices such as prayer, meditation, and contemplation, we can activate the pineal gland and deepen our spiritual connection, leading to profound insights and enlightenment.

Pineal Gland Supplements and Natural Remedies for Enhancing its Function:

Certain supplements and natural remedies, such as melatonin, ashwagandha, and certain essential oils, can support the pineal gland's function and stimulate psychic abilities and intuition. However, it is essential to consult with a healthcare professional before incorporating any new supplements into your routine.

Pineal Gland and its Relationship with Lucid Dreaming and Astral Projection:

The pineal gland is closely associated with lucid dreaming and astral projection, allowing us to explore different realms and dimensions. By practicing techniques like dream journaling, reality checks, and astral projection exercises, we can harness the power of the pineal gland and unlock these extraordinary experiences.

Pineal Gland and its Significance in Ancient and Alternative Healing Practices:

Throughout history, various ancient and alternative healing practices have recognized the importance of the pineal gland in promoting overall well-being. Techniques such as acupuncture, energy healing, and sound therapy can activate and balance the pineal gland, facilitating the development of psychic abilities and intuition.

Pineal Gland and its Role in Psychic Abilities and Intuition Development:

The pineal gland acts as a conduit for psychic abilities and intuition. By practicing visualization, remote viewing, and psychic exercises, we can strengthen our connection to this gland and enhance our innate psychic potential.

Pineal Gland and its Association with the Third Eye Chakra and Energy Healing:

The pineal gland is closely associated with the third eye chakra, which is the energetic center responsible for intuition and clairvoyance. Through energy healing practices like Reiki, crystal healing, and chakra balancing, we can stimulate and activate the pineal gland, promoting psychic abilities and intuition.

Pineal Gland and its Impact on Mood, Emotions, and Mental Well-being:

The pineal gland influences our mood, emotions, and overall mental well-being. By maintaining a healthy lifestyle, managing stress levels, and incorporating relaxation techniques like yoga and deep breathing, we can support the pineal gland's optimal function and enhance our psychic abilities and intuition.

In conclusion, by understanding the techniques for developing psychic abilities and intuition and their connection to the pineal gland, we can embark on a transformative journey of self-discovery and spiritual growth. With dedication, practice, and a holistic approach to well-being, we can unlock the full potential of our minds and connect with the profound wisdom that lies within us.

# Chapter 10: The Pineal Gland and its Association with the Third Eye Chakra and Energy Healing

Understanding the Third Eye Chakra

The third eye chakra is a topic that has gained significant attention in recent years, particularly in the realms of spirituality and energy healing. In order to truly comprehend the significance of this chakra, it is essential to understand its connection with the pineal gland.

The third eye chakra, also known as Ajna, is located in the middle of the forehead, just above the space between the eyebrows. It is associated with intuition, insight, and spiritual awareness. This chakra acts as a gateway to higher consciousness, allowing individuals to tap into their inner wisdom and connect with the divine.

The pineal gland, a small gland located deep within the brain, is believed to be the physical manifestation of the third eye chakra. It is responsible for the synthesis and secretion of melatonin, a hormone that regulates sleep and wakefulness. Furthermore, the pineal gland is associated with the production of dimethyltryptamine (DMT), a naturally occurring psychedelic compound that is thought to facilitate spiritual experiences and altered states of consciousness.

When the third eye chakra is balanced and open, individuals may experience enhanced intuition, clarity of thought, and a deeper connection to their inner selves. They may also develop psychic abilities, such as clairvoyance or telepathy, and experience a heightened sense of spiritual awakening and enlightenment.

There are various techniques that can be employed to activate and balance the third eye chakra. Meditation and mindfulness practices are particularly effective in this regard. By quieting the mind and focusing inward, individuals can stimulate the flow of energy to the third eye chakra, thereby expanding their awareness and enhancing their spiritual growth.

In addition to meditation, certain natural remedies and supplements can also support the function of the pineal gland and the third eye chakra. These include herbs like ashwagandha, passionflower, and ginkgo biloba, as well as essential oils like frankincense and sandalwood. However, it is important to consult with a healthcare professional before incorporating any new supplements into your routine.

The third eye chakra and the pineal gland are also closely connected to sleep and circadian rhythm regulation. By maintaining a healthy sleep schedule and engaging in practices that promote deep rest, individuals can support the optimal functioning of their third eye chakra and enhance their overall mental well-being.

In conclusion, the third eye chakra and its connection with the pineal gland play a significant role in our mental well-being and spiritual growth. By understanding and nurturing this chakra, individuals can tap into their innate intuition, develop their psychic abilities, and experience a profound sense of spiritual awakening and enlightenment.

The Pineal Gland's Relationship with Energy Healing

Energy healing is a fascinating and increasingly popular approach to holistic well-being that recognizes the interconnectedness of the mind, body, and spirit. In recent years, there has been a growing interest in the role of the pineal gland in energy healing practices. This subchapter explores the profound relationship between the pineal gland and energy healing, shedding light on its impact on mental well-being and overall health.

One of the key aspects of the pineal gland's connection with energy healing is its role in regulating the body's energy centers, often referred to as chakras. The pineal gland is believed to be closely associated with the third eye chakra, which is considered the gateway to higher consciousness and spiritual awakening. By activating and balancing the third eye chakra, individuals can tap into their intuition, psychic abilities, and spiritual insights, enhancing their energy healing practices.

Furthermore, the pineal gland is known to produce and release melatonin, a hormone that regulates sleep and wakefulness. This hormone plays a crucial role in maintaining our circadian rhythm, the internal clock that governs our sleep-wake cycle. Energy healing techniques, such as meditation and mindfulness, have been found to stimulate the pineal gland, leading to the production of melatonin and promoting restful sleep. Adequate sleep is essential for optimal mental well-being, and the pineal gland plays a significant role in ensuring a healthy sleep pattern.

The pineal gland is also deeply intertwined with ancient and alternative healing practices. Many traditional healing modalities, such as Ayurveda and Traditional Chinese Medicine, recognize the pineal gland's significance in maintaining overall health and vitality. Certain herbs, supplements, and natural remedies are believed to enhance the function of the pineal gland and promote its optimal performance. These remedies include practices like pineal gland detoxification techniques and the use of specific herbs like ashwagandha and holy basil.

Moreover, the pineal gland's relationship with energy healing extends to the realm of lucid dreaming and astral projection. Lucid dreaming is the ability to consciously control and navigate dreams, while astral projection refers to the out-of-body experiences in which one's consciousness leaves the physical body. These experiences are closely associated with the pineal gland, as it is believed to facilitate the connection between the physical and spiritual realms.

In conclusion, the pineal gland's relationship with energy healing is multifaceted and profound. From its role in regulating sleep and circadian rhythms to its connection with spiritual awakening and intuition development, the pineal gland plays a crucial role in enhancing mental well-being and overall health. By understanding and harnessing the power of the pineal gland, individuals can unlock their full potential for healing, growth, and spiritual enlightenment.

Practices for Balancing and Activating the Third Eye Chakra

The third eye chakra, also known as the Ajna chakra, is closely associated with the pineal gland. Located in the center of the forehead, this chakra is believed to be the gateway to higher consciousness, psychic abilities, and spiritual awakening. When balanced and activated, the third eye chakra can enhance intuition, improve mental clarity, and promote a deep sense of inner knowing.

To support the health and vitality of your third eye chakra, here are some practices you can incorporate into your daily routine:

1. Meditation and Mindfulness: Regular meditation practice is one of the most effective ways to activate and balance the third eye chakra. Find a quiet and comfortable space, close your eyes, and focus your attention on the area between your eyebrows. Visualize a deep indigo or purple light radiating from within, energizing and opening your third eye.

2. Breathwork: Deep, conscious breathing can help clear any energetic blockages in your third eye chakra. Take slow, deep breaths in through your nose, and exhale through your mouth, visualizing any negativity or tension leaving your body with each breath.

3. Yoga Poses: Certain yoga poses can stimulate and activate the third eye chakra. Poses like child's pose, downward facing dog, and seated forward fold gently open the energy channels in the body, allowing for a free flow of energy to the third eye.

4. Crystal Healing: Crystals such as amethyst, lapis lazuli, and clear quartz are known to support the third eye chakra. Place these crystals on your forehead during meditation or wear them as jewelry to enhance and balance the energy of your third eye.

5. Affirmations: Practice affirmations that are specifically designed to activate and balance the third eye chakra. Repeat statements such as "I trust my intuition," "I see clearly and trust my inner guidance," or "I am open to receiving divine wisdom" to align your thoughts and beliefs with the energy of your third eye.

By incorporating these practices into your daily routine, you can begin to balance and activate your third eye chakra. As you cultivate a deeper connection with your intuition and inner wisdom, you may experience a greater sense of clarity, spiritual growth, and enhanced mental well-being. Remember to always listen to your body and intuition, and adjust these practices to suit your unique needs and preferences.

# Chapter 11: The Pineal Gland and its Impact on Mood, Emotions, and Mental Well-being

How the Pineal Gland Influences Mood and Emotions

The pineal gland, a small endocrine gland located deep within the brain, is often referred to as the "third eye" due to its association with spiritual enlightenment and intuition. However, its influence extends far beyond just these aspects. In fact, the pineal gland plays a crucial role in regulating our mood, emotions, and overall mental well-being.

One of the key ways in which the pineal gland influences mood and emotions is through the production and secretion of melatonin. Melatonin is a hormone that helps regulate our sleep-wake cycle, also known as our circadian rhythm. When the pineal gland releases melatonin, it signals to our body that it's time to sleep, promoting a sense of relaxation and calmness. Consequently, a disruption in melatonin production can lead to sleep disorders such as insomnia, which in turn can have a negative impact on our mood and emotions.

Furthermore, the pineal gland is closely connected to the production of serotonin, a neurotransmitter that is often referred to as the "feel-good" hormone. Serotonin is responsible for regulating our mood, appetite, and sleep patterns. Low levels of serotonin have been associated with depression and anxiety, while higher levels promote feelings of happiness and well-being. The pineal gland plays a crucial role in the synthesis of serotonin, highlighting its significance in maintaining a balanced mood.

In addition to its role in hormone production, the pineal gland is also connected to our spiritual and intuitive experiences. Many ancient and alternative healing practices attribute the pineal gland as the gateway to higher consciousness and spiritual awakening. Through practices such as meditation and mindfulness, individuals can activate and enhance the function of the pineal gland, leading to a heightened sense of awareness, intuition, and overall mental well-being.

Moreover, the pineal gland's association with the third eye chakra, an energy center located in the middle of the forehead, further emphasizes its impact on our mood and emotions. The third eye chakra is believed to be the center of intuition and higher perception. By balancing and activating the pineal gland, individuals can tap into their innate psychic abilities and develop a deeper connection with their emotions, leading to improved mental well-being.

While there are various techniques and practices available to enhance pineal gland function, it is important to note that natural remedies and supplements can also support its optimal performance. Certain herbs and nutrients, such as ashwagandha, turmeric, and vitamin D, have been shown to nourish and stimulate the pineal gland, thereby promoting a healthy mood and emotional balance.

In conclusion, the pineal gland plays a vital role in influencing our mood, emotions, and overall mental well-being. Through its regulation of hormones such as melatonin and serotonin, as well as its connection to spirituality and intuition, the pineal gland is a key player in maintaining a balanced and joyful state of mind. By understanding and utilizing techniques to detoxify, activate, and enhance the function of the pineal gland, individuals can unlock their full potential for emotional well-being and spiritual growth.

Strategies for Maintaining Mental Well-being through Pineal Gland Care

In this subchapter, we will explore various strategies for maintaining mental well-being through the care of the pineal gland. The pineal gland, often referred to as the "third eye," plays a crucial role in our mental and emotional health, as well as our spiritual development. By understanding how to care for and support the pineal gland, we can enhance our overall mental well-being.

One essential strategy for pineal gland care is through pineal gland detoxification techniques. Over time, the pineal gland can become calcified due to exposure to toxins from our environment and diet. Detoxification practices, such as adopting a clean and organic diet, avoiding fluoride-containing products, and incorporating specific herbs and supplements, can help remove these toxins and restore the pineal gland's optimal functioning.

Another powerful strategy is pineal gland activation through meditation and mindfulness. By incorporating regular meditation practices that focus on the third eye region, we can stimulate and activate the pineal gland. This activation can lead to heightened states of consciousness, increased intuition, and a deeper connection to our spiritual selves.

Understanding the pineal gland's role in sleep and circadian rhythm regulation is also crucial for maintaining mental well-being. By ensuring a healthy sleep routine and creating a sleep environment that supports pineal gland function, we can improve our sleep quality and overall mental health. This can involve practices such as maintaining a consistent sleep schedule, limiting exposure to blue light before bed, and creating a relaxing sleep environment.

Exploring the pineal gland's connection with spiritual awakening and enlightenment is another important aspect of maintaining mental well-being. By nurturing our spiritual selves through practices like meditation, energy healing, and connecting with nature, we can experience a profound sense of purpose, inner peace, and fulfillment.

Additionally, incorporating pineal gland supplements and natural remedies can enhance its function. Certain supplements, such as melatonin, vitamin D, and specific herbs like ashwagandha and holy basil, can support pineal gland health and promote mental well-being.

Understanding the pineal gland's role in lucid dreaming and astral projection can also be beneficial for mental well-being. By exploring these practices, we can tap into our subconscious mind, expand our awareness, and gain valuable insights and experiences that contribute to our overall mental health.

Recognizing the significance of the pineal gland in ancient and alternative healing practices is essential. Various traditional healing modalities, such as Ayurveda and Chinese medicine, have long recognized the importance of the pineal gland in balancing the body, mind, and spirit.

Furthermore, the pineal gland's role in psychic abilities and intuition development should not be overlooked. By practicing mindfulness, meditation, and energy healing techniques, we can cultivate and enhance our intuitive abilities, leading to a heightened sense of awareness and mental well-being.

Lastly, understanding the pineal gland's association with the third eye chakra and energy healing can provide valuable insights into maintaining mental well-being. By balancing and harmonizing the third eye chakra through practices such as yoga, Reiki, and crystal healing, we can promote mental clarity, intuition, and emotional well-being.

In conclusion, by implementing these strategies for maintaining mental well-being through pineal gland care, we can enhance our overall mental health, emotional balance, and spiritual growth. The pineal gland plays a vital role in our well-being, and by nurturing and supporting its function, we can experience a profound transformation in our lives.

Integrating Pineal Gland Support into a Holistic Mental Health Approach

The pineal gland, a small pea-sized gland located in the center of the brain, has long been associated with spiritual and metaphysical experiences. However, recent scientific research has shed light on its crucial role in mental well-being and overall health. In this subchapter, we will explore how integrating pineal gland support into a holistic mental health approach can enhance our overall well-being.

One of the key aspects of pineal gland support is detoxification techniques. Toxins from our environment and diet can accumulate in the pineal gland, impairing its function. Implementing detoxification practices such as consuming organic foods, avoiding chemicals, and using natural personal care products can help cleanse the pineal gland and optimize its performance.

Another effective way to support the pineal gland is through meditation and mindfulness. By practicing regular meditation, we can calm the mind, reduce stress, and activate the pineal gland. Mindfulness techniques, such as focusing on the present moment and maintaining awareness, can also help us connect with our pineal gland and tap into its potential.

The pineal gland plays a vital role in sleep and circadian rhythm regulation. It produces melatonin, a hormone that regulates our sleep-wake cycle. By prioritizing good sleep hygiene practices, such as establishing a consistent sleep schedule and creating a relaxing bedtime routine, we can support the pineal gland's natural production of melatonin and improve our sleep quality.

Moreover, the pineal gland has been associated with spiritual awakening and enlightenment. Through various practices like meditation, yoga, and breathwork, we can activate the pineal gland and experience heightened spiritual states. These practices can open the doorway to a deeper understanding of ourselves and the world around us.

Additionally, certain supplements and natural remedies can enhance the function of the pineal gland. Substances like melatonin, 5-HTP, and certain herbs like ashwagandha and bacopa have been shown to support pineal gland health. However, it is important to consult with a healthcare professional before incorporating any supplements into your routine.

The pineal gland also plays a role in lucid dreaming and astral projection. By maintaining a healthy pineal gland and practicing techniques like dream journaling, reality checks, and lucid dreaming induction methods, we can enhance our dream experiences and explore the depths of our consciousness.

Furthermore, ancient and alternative healing practices have long recognized the significance of the pineal gland. Modalities like Ayurveda, Traditional Chinese Medicine, and indigenous healing traditions often incorporate techniques that support the pineal gland's function, such as herbal remedies, sound healing, and energy work.

The pineal gland is closely associated with psychic abilities and intuition development. By honing our intuitive skills through practices like meditation, energy healing, and divination, we can strengthen the connection with our pineal gland and tap into our innate psychic potential.

In addition, the pineal gland is often linked to the third eye chakra, an energy center located between the eyebrows. Through energy healing modalities like Reiki and chakra balancing, we can activate and balance the third eye chakra, promoting overall energetic well-being.

Finally, the pineal gland's impact on mood, emotions, and mental well-being cannot be overlooked. Imbalances in the pineal gland can contribute to mood disorders, anxiety, and depression. By adopting a holistic approach that includes healthy lifestyle habits, stress management techniques, and emotional healing practices, we can support the pineal gland and improve our mental well-being.

In conclusion, integrating pineal gland support into a holistic mental health approach holds tremendous potential for enhancing our overall well-being. By implementing detoxification techniques, practicing meditation and mindfulness, prioritizing sleep, exploring spirituality, utilizing supplements and natural remedies, embracing lucid dreaming and astral projection, incorporating ancient healing practices, developing psychic abilities, balancing the third eye chakra, and prioritizing mental well-being, we can unlock the full potential of the pineal gland and experience a profound transformation in our lives.

Conclusion: Harnessing the Power of the Mind-Body Connection through the Pineal Gland

Throughout this book, we have delved into the fascinating world of the pineal gland and its profound impact on our mental well-being. The pineal gland, often referred to as the "third eye," holds immense potential for our overall health, consciousness, and spiritual growth. In this concluding chapter, we will summarize the key insights we have gained and explore the ways in which we can harness the power of the mind-body connection through the pineal gland.

Firstly, we have learned about various pineal gland detoxification techniques. By adopting a healthy lifestyle, practicing regular exercise, and incorporating detoxifying foods into our diet, we can support the optimal functioning of the pineal gland. Detoxification helps to remove harmful substances and toxins that may hinder the pineal gland's ability to regulate our mental well-being.

Next, we explored the importance of meditation and mindfulness in activating the pineal gland. Through these practices, we can calm our minds, enhance our focus, and strengthen our connection with the pineal gland. By incorporating meditation and mindfulness into our daily routines, we can tap into the immense potential of our pineal gland, leading to increased clarity, intuition, and spiritual awakening.

Furthermore, we have discovered the vital role of the pineal gland in sleep and circadian rhythm regulation. By maintaining a healthy sleep schedule, avoiding artificial light, and creating a conducive sleep environment, we can optimize the pineal gland's production of melatonin, a hormone that regulates sleep patterns. This, in turn, promotes improved sleep quality and overall mental well-being.

We have also explored the pineal gland's connection with spiritual awakening and enlightenment. Through practices such as yoga, breathwork, and exploring our consciousness, we can awaken the dormant potential within the pineal gland. This can lead to profound spiritual experiences, expanded awareness, and a deeper understanding of ourselves and the world around us.

Additionally, we have examined the role of natural remedies and supplements in enhancing the pineal gland's function. Certain herbs, such as ashwagandha and ginkgo biloba, along with supplements like melatonin and magnesium, can support the pineal gland and promote its optimal performance. However, it is essential to consult with a healthcare professional before incorporating any supplements into our routine.

Moreover, we have explored the pineal gland's association with lucid dreaming, astral projection, psychic abilities, and intuition development. By honing our awareness and practicing specific techniques, we can tap into the pineal gland's ability to access higher realms of consciousness and unlock our innate psychic capabilities.

Furthermore, we have discussed the significance of the pineal gland in ancient and alternative healing practices. From Ayurveda to Traditional

Chinese Medicine, various ancient cultures recognized the pineal gland's vital role in overall health and well-being. By incorporating these alternative healing practices into our lives, we can support the pineal gland and promote holistic healing.

Lastly, we have examined the pineal gland's impact on mood, emotions, and mental well-being. Imbalances in the pineal gland can lead to mood disorders, such as depression and anxiety. By adopting strategies to support the pineal gland, such as sunlight exposure, stress reduction techniques, and a healthy diet, we can cultivate emotional balance and enhance our mental well-being.

In conclusion, the pineal gland holds tremendous power in influencing our mental well-being, consciousness, and spiritual growth. By understanding and harnessing the mind-body connection through the pineal gland, we can unlock our full potential, achieve optimal mental health, and embark on a transformative journey towards enlightenment and self-discovery.

www.ingramcontent.com/pod-product-compliance
Lightning Source LLC
Chambersburg PA
CBHW031414160726
47993CB00003B/1228